Birth without Violence

FRÉDÉRICK LEBOYER

New translation by Yvonne Fitzgerald

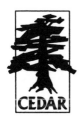

CEDAR

A Mandarin Paperback
BIRTH WITHOUT VIOLENCE

First published in Great Britain 1975
by Wildwood House Ltd
This revised edition published 1991
by Mandarin Paperbacks
an imprint of Reed International Books Ltd
Michelin House, 81 Fulham Road, London SW3 6RB
and Auckland, Melbourne, Singapore and Toronto
Reissued 1993, 1995 by Cedar

Originally published in France as
Pour Une Naissance Sans Violence
by Editions du Seuil, Paris.
Copyright © 1974 by Editions du Seuil
Translation copyright © 1990 by Alfred A. Knopf, Inc.

All the photographs were taken
by Frédérick Leboyer and Pierre Marie Goulet
except for those on pages 14, 17 and 28,
which were supplied by I.M.S. Stockholm.

A CIP catalogue record for this title
is available from the British Library
ISBN 0 7493 0642 4

Printed in England by Clays Ltd, St Ives plc